Balanced Bites

A Guide to Sustaining Your Ideal Shape

Stephanie C. Levine

Copyright

Table Of Content

Introduction

Welcome to "Balanced Bites: A Guide to Sustaining Your Ideal Shape." In today's fast-paced world, the quest for our ideal shape often feels like an endless pursuit, fraught with frustration and disappointment. We're bombarded with promises of quick fixes and drastic transformations, only to find ourselves right back where we started, if not worse off than before.

But what if I told you that achieving and maintaining your ideal shape doesn't have to be a battle? What if I told you that you could nourish your body, enjoy your food, and feel great in your skin—all without resorting to extreme measures or deprivation? That's precisely what "Balanced Bites" is all about. This book isn't just another diet plan for a weight loss program. It's a holistic approach to health and wellness that recognizes the interconnectedness of our physical, mental, and emotional well-being. "Balanced Bites" offers a roadmap for creating sustainable habits that support your long-term health goals. From understanding the fundamentals of nutrition to developing a positive mindset around food and body image, each chapter is packed with practical insights and actionable strategies to assist you in developing a better connection with food and with yourself.

But "Balanced Bites" is more than just a collection of information—it's a journey of self-discovery and empowerment. As you delve into its pages, you'll learn to tune into your body's hunger and fullness cues, experiment with new flavors and ingredients, and cultivate a deeper sense of mindfulness around eating. You'll discover that achieving your ideal shape is not just about what you eat, but how you eat and how you live. And because life is too short to eat boring food, "Balanced Bites" also features a mouthwatering selection of recipes that prove healthy eating can be delicious, satisfying, and downright enjoyable. From vibrant salads and hearty soups to indulgent desserts and everything in between, these recipes are designed to nourish your body and tantalize your taste buds, all while supporting your health and wellness goals.

So if you're tired of yo-yo dieting, unsustainable meal plans, and feeling at war with your body, it's time to embrace a new approach. It's time to say goodbye to extremes and hello to balance.

It's time to reclaim your health, your happiness, and your ideal shape with "Balanced Bites" as your guide. Let's embark on this journey together, one bite at a time.

Chapter 1
Understanding Your Body

In our journey towards sustaining our ideal shape, it's crucial to begin by understanding our bodies from within. This chapter delves into three key aspects: Body Composition, Metabolism, and Genetics and Body Shape.

1. Body Composition

Body composition refers to the ratio of fat to lean tissue in our bodies. Understanding our body composition provides insight into our overall health and fitness levels. While fat is essential for various bodily functions, excess fat can lead to health issues. By assessing and managing our body composition, we can strive for a healthier balance that supports our ideal shape.Body composition encompasses more than just body weight; it includes the distribution of fat and lean mass throughout the body. Lean mass consists of muscles, bones, organs, and tissues, while fat mass refers to adipose tissue. Understanding body composition is vital because it affects overall health and fitness.

A. Fat Distribution:

Different areas of the body store fat differently, and where fat accumulates can impact health risks. For example, visceral fat stored around organs poses greater health risks than subcutaneous fat stored just beneath the skin.

B. Lean Body Mass:

Building and preserving lean muscle mass is essential for metabolic health, strength, and functionality. Resistance training and adequate protein intake are crucial for maintaining lean body mass.

C. **Body Fat Percentage:**

Monitoring body fat percentage provides a more accurate assessment of health and fitness than body weight alone. It reflects the proportion of fat mass to total body weight and can be measured using various methods such as skinfold calipers, bioelectrical impedance analysis, or dual-energy X-ray absorptiometry (DEXA).

2. Metabolism

The process by which our bodies turn food and liquids into energy is called metabolism. It's influenced by factors such as age, gender, muscle mass, and physical activity level.

Understanding our metabolism helps us make informed decisions about nutrition and exercise. By optimizing our metabolism, we can better maintain our ideal shape and energy levels.Metabolism is the sum of all biochemical processes that occur within the body to sustain life. Several factors influence metabolism, including:

A. Basal Metabolic Rate (BMR):
BMR is the number of calories your body needs to maintain basic physiological functions at rest. Age, gender, heredity, and body composition are a few examples of factors that affect BMR. Strength training is a good way to increase muscle mass and increase BMR.

B. Thermic Effect of Food (TEF):

TEF refers to the energy expended during digestion, absorption, and metabolism of nutrients from food. The biggest thermic impact is seen in protein, which is followed by lipids and carbs.

C. **Physical Activity Level (PAL):**

PAL accounts for the energy expended through physical activity and exercise. Regular exercise, including both cardiovascular and strength training, can increase calorie expenditure and improve metabolic health.

3. **Genetics and Body Shape**

Our genetics play a significant role in determining our body shape and size. While we can't change our genetics, we can work with them to achieve our desired physique.

Understanding our genetic predispositions empowers us to set realistic goals and tailor our lifestyle choices accordingly. By embracing our unique genetic makeup, we can work towards sustaining our ideal shape healthily and sustainably.Our genetic makeup influences various aspects of body composition, metabolism, and body shape:

A. Body Type:

Genetics contribute to determining our body types, such as ectomorph, mesomorph, or endomorph. While genetics may predispose individuals to certain body types, lifestyle factors like diet and exercise can still significantly impact body composition.

B. Fat Storage Patterns:

Genetic factors influence where fat is stored in the body. Some individuals may tend to store excess fat in specific areas, such as the abdomen or hips, based on genetic predispositions.

C. **Metabolic Rate:**

Genetic variations can affect metabolic rate and how efficiently the body processes and utilizes nutrients. While genetic factors play a role, lifestyle choices such as diet, exercise, and sleep quality also influence metabolic health.

Understanding our body composition, metabolism, and genetic predispositions lays the foundation for sustaining our ideal shape. By gaining insights into these aspects, we can make informed choices that support our health and well-being. In the chapters ahead, we'll explore practical strategies and techniques to help us achieve and maintain our balanced bites.

Chapter 2
Nutrition Fundamentals

In this chapter, we'll delve into the essential elements of nutrition that form the foundation of sustaining your ideal shape. Understanding macronutrients, micronutrients, and the significance of balanced eating is crucial for achieving and maintaining your desired physique.

1. Macronutrients:

The nutrients that our bodies need in substantial quantities in order to function at their best are known as macronutrients.They are divided into three main categories:

A. Carbohydrates:

Carbohydrates are the body's primary source of energy. They provide fuel for daily activities and exercise. Complex carbohydrates found in whole grains, fruits, and vegetables offer sustained energy release, while simple carbohydrates like sugars provide quick bursts of energy. Balancing your carbohydrate intake is essential to prevent energy spikes and crashes.

B. Proteins:

Proteins are the building blocks of our body tissues, including muscles, bones, skin, and organs. They are necessary for maintaining, growing, and repairing muscles. Meat, poultry, fish, eggs, dairy products, legumes, and nuts are examples of dietary protein sources. Eating enough protein promotes satiety, which reduces appetite and aids in the development of muscles.

C. Fats:

Fats are vital for various bodily functions, including hormone production, absorption of fat-soluble vitamins, and insulation of organs. Healthy fats, such as those found in avocados, nuts, seeds, olive oil, and fatty fish, should comprise the majority of your fat intake. Limiting saturated and trans fats from processed and fried foods is essential for heart health and weight management.

2. Micronutrients:

While macronutrients provide energy and structural components, micronutrients are essential for regulating metabolism, supporting immune function, and maintaining overall health. Micronutrients include vitamins and minerals, and each plays a unique role in the body:

A. Vitamins:

These organic compounds are required in small amounts but are crucial for various physiological functions. For example, vitamin C supports immune health, vitamin D aids in calcium absorption for bone health, and the B-complex vitamins are involved in energy metabolism. Consuming a diverse array of fruits, vegetables, whole grains, and lean proteins ensures adequate vitamin intake.

B. Minerals:

Minerals are inorganic substances that are essential for numerous physiological processes, such as bone formation, fluid balance, and nerve function. Calcium, magnesium, potassium, iron, and zinc are among the essential minerals needed for optimal health. Consuming a balanced diet rich in whole foods ensures sufficient mineral intake.

Importance of Balanced Eating

Balanced eating involves consuming a variety of nutrient-dense foods in appropriate portions to meet your body's needs while maintaining energy balance. Here's why it's crucial:

A. Optimal Nutrient Intake:
Eating a variety of foods ensures you obtain all the essential nutrients your body needs for proper functioning.

B. Weight Management:

Balancing macronutrients helps regulate appetite and prevent overeating, leading to better weight management and body composition.

C. Energy Levels:

Consuming a balanced diet provides sustained energy throughout the day, reducing fatigue and improving productivity.

D. Disease Prevention:

A balanced diet rich in fruits, vegetables, whole grains, lean proteins, and healthy fats can reduce the risk of chronic diseases such as heart disease, diabetes, and certain cancers.

E. Overall Well-being:

Proper nutrition supports mental clarity, mood stability, and overall well-being, enhancing your quality of life.

By understanding and implementing the principles of balanced eating, you can sustain your ideal shape while promoting long-term health and vitality. In the following chapters, we'll explore practical strategies and tips for incorporating balanced nutrition into your daily life.

Chapter 3
Designing Your Balanced Plate

In this chapter, we delve into the intricacies of creating a balanced plate that not only sustains your ideal shape but also supports overall well-being. We'll explore the importance of portion control, how to build balanced meals, and foster healthy eating habits for long-term success.

1. **Portion Control**:

Portion control is the cornerstone of maintaining a healthy weight and achieving nutritional balance. It involves being mindful of the amount of food you consume, rather than relying solely on what you eat. Here's a detailed breakdown:

A. Understanding Serving Sizes:

Begin by familiarizing yourself with standard serving sizes for different food groups. Tools like measuring cups, food scales, or visual references (like a deck of cards for protein) can aid in portion estimation.

B. Listen to Your Body:

Pay attention to hunger and satiety cues. Eat slowly, savoring each bite, and stop when you feel comfortably satisfied, not overly full.

C. Practice Moderation:

Enjoying occasional treats is fine, but be mindful of portion sizes. Opt for smaller servings of high-calorie or indulgent foods to keep your overall intake in check.

2. Building Balanced Meals:

A balanced meal incorporates a variety of nutrients to support overall health and energy levels. Here's how to construct one:

A. Include Lean Proteins:

Protein is essential for muscle repair, metabolism, and satiety. Incorporate lean sources like poultry, fish, tofu, beans, or lentils into each meal.

B. Add Whole Grains:

Whole grains provide fiber, vitamins, and minerals. Opt for options like brown rice, quinoa, whole wheat pasta, or oats to promote sustained energy levels and digestive health.

C. Load Up on Vegetables:

Try to have colorful vegetables make up half of your plate.They're low in calories but high in fiber, antioxidants, and essential nutrients. Experiment with different cooking methods and seasonings to enhance flavor.

D. Incorporate Healthy Fats:

Don't shy away from fats; just choose the right kinds. Include sources like avocados, nuts, seeds, and olive oil for heart-healthy fats that support brain function and nutrient absorption.

E. Don't Forget Calcium:

Incorporate dairy or fortified alternatives like almond milk or tofu to meet calcium needs for strong bones and teeth.

3. Healthy Eating Habits:

Sustaining your ideal shape goes beyond just what's on your plate; it's also about cultivating healthy eating habits. Here's how to foster them:

A. Mindful Eating:

Practice mindful eating by focusing on the sensory experience of each meal. Turn off distractions, chew slowly, and savor the flavors and textures of your food.

B. Plan Ahead:

Plan your meals and snacks ahead of time to avoid impulsive choices or reaching for convenience foods. Batch cooking and meal prepping can streamline the process and ensure nutritious options are readily available.

C. Stay Hydrated:

Drink plenty of water throughout the day to stay hydrated and stave off hunger cues that may be mistaken for thirst.

D. **Manage Stress**:

Stress can impact eating behaviors and food choices. Incorporate stress-relieving activities like meditation, yoga, or deep breathing exercises into your routine to support overall well-being.

By implementing these strategies for portion control, building balanced meals, and cultivating healthy eating habits, you'll not only sustain your ideal shape but also enhance your overall quality of life. Remember, it's about progress, not perfection, so be patient and consistent in your efforts toward optimal health and vitality.

Chapter 4
The Role of Exercise

In this chapter, we'll delve into the crucial role that exercise plays in maintaining a balanced and healthy lifestyle. We'll explore various types of exercises, how to create an effective fitness routine, and tailor exercises to your specific body shape.

1. Types of Exercise

A. Cardiovascular Exercise:

Cardio workouts, such as running, cycling, or swimming, are excellent for improving heart health, burning calories, and increasing endurance.

B. Strength Training:

Strength training involves resistance exercises like weightlifting or bodyweight exercises. It helps build muscle mass, boost metabolism, and improve overall strength and stability.

C. Flexibility and Mobility:

Activities like yoga, Pilates, or stretching routines enhance flexibility, mobility, and posture. They also reduce the risk of injuries and promote relaxation.

D. Balance and Stability:

Exercises that focus on balance and stability, such as tai chi or stability ball workouts, help improve coordination and prevent falls, especially as we age.

2. Creating a Fitness Routine

A. **Set Clear Goals**:

Determine what you want to achieve with your exercise routine, whether it's weight loss, muscle gain, improved endurance, or overall health.

B. **Choose Activities You Enjoy:**

Find exercises that you genuinely enjoy, as this increases adherence to your routine. It could be dancing, hiking, or playing a sport.

C. **Start Slowly and Progress Gradually:**

Begin with manageable intensity and duration, then gradually increase as your fitness improves to avoid burnout or injury.

D. **Incorporate Variety:**

Include a mix of cardiovascular, strength, flexibility, and balance exercises to ensure a well-rounded routine and prevent boredom.

E. Schedule Regular Workouts:

Consistency is key to seeing results. Set aside specific times for exercise in your weekly schedule and treat them as non-negotiable appointments.

F. Listen to Your Body:

Pay attention to how your body responds to exercise. Rest when needed, and don't push through pain or discomfort that could lead to injury.

3. Exercise for Your Body Shape

A. Ectomorphs:

Individuals with a naturally lean and slender build may focus on strength training to add muscle mass and shape to their frame. Compound exercises like squats, deadlifts, and bench presses are beneficial.

B. Mesomorphs:

Those with a muscular and well-proportioned body type can engage in a balanced mix of strength training and cardiovascular exercise to maintain their physique. They may also enjoy activities like HIIT (High-Intensity Interval Training) for optimal results.

C. Endomorphs:

People with a rounder and softer physique may benefit from a combination of strength training, cardio, and flexibility exercises to manage body fat and build lean muscle. Focus on consistency and gradually increasing intensity.

By understanding the various types of exercises, creating a personalized fitness routine, and tailoring workouts to your body shape, you'll be well-equipped to sustain your ideal shape and enjoy a healthier, more balanced lifestyle. Remember, consistency and patience are key on this journey towards optimal well-being.

Chapter 5
Mindful Eating

In this chapter, we delve into the concept of mindful eating, a practice that goes beyond just what we eat, focusing on how we eat and our relationship with food. By becoming more mindful of our eating habits, we can better sustain our ideal shape by fostering a healthier relationship with food.

1. Listening to Your Body:

Mindful eating starts with tuning into your body's hunger and fullness cues. Many of us have lost touch with these signals due to busy lifestyles, emotional eating, or external influences. Here's how you can reconnect with your body:

A. Pause before Eating:

Before every meal or snack, take a moment to check in with your body. Are you truly hungry, or are you eating out of habit or emotion?

B. Eat Slowly:

Chew your food thoroughly and savor each bite. Eating slowly allows your body to register fullness more accurately, preventing overeating.

C. **Check-in During Meals**:

Throughout your meal, periodically pause and assess your hunger levels. Even if there is food left on your plate, you should stop eating when you are satisfied.

D. Mindful Snacking:

Apply the same principles of mindful eating to snacks. Before reaching for a snack, ask yourself if you're truly hungry or if you're eating out of boredom or stress.

2. Overcoming Emotional Eating:

Emotional eating frequently stands in the way of upholding a healthy diet and perfect form.Many of us turn to food for comfort, stress relief, or as a coping mechanism. Here's how to address emotional eating:

A. **Identify Triggers**:

Pay attention to the emotions and situations that trigger your desire to eat. Maintain a food journal to monitor your eating habits and the feelings that go along with them.

B. Develop Coping Strategies:

Instead of turning to food, find alternative ways to cope with emotions such as stress, boredom, or sadness. This could include practicing mindfulness, exercising, journaling, or talking to a friend.

C. Practice Self-Compassion:

Be kind to yourself when you slip up.Recommit to your mindful eating objectives and accept your emotional eating as a teaching opportunity rather than criticizing yourself for it.

D. Seek Professional Support:

If emotional eating is a persistent challenge for you, consider seeking support from a therapist or counselor who specializes in emotional eating or disordered eating behaviors. Therapy can provide you with personalized strategies and tools to address the underlying emotions driving your eating habits.

E. Practice Stress Management Techniques:

Since stress is a common trigger for emotional eating, learning stress management techniques can help you cope with emotions in healthier ways. Techniques such as deep breathing exercises, meditation, yoga, or progressive muscle relaxation can help you relax and reduce stress levels, reducing the likelihood of turning to food for comfort

3. Strategies for Mindful Eating:

A. Remove Distractions:

Turn off the TV, put away your phone, and focus solely on the act of eating. Distractions can lead to mindless overeating.

B. **Use All Your Senses**:

Engage all your senses while eating. Take note of your food's flavors, textures, colors, and scents.This can enhance the eating experience and satisfaction.

C. **Portion Control**:

Be mindful of portion sizes.If you want to help regulate portion sizes and avoid overeating, use smaller dishes and plates.

D. **Practice Gratitude:**

Before each meal, take a moment to express gratitude for the food you are about to eat. This

can help cultivate a positive relationship with
food and promote mindful eating.

By incorporating these strategies into your daily
routine, you can cultivate a healthier relationship
with food and sustain your ideal shape for the
long term. Mindful eating isn't just about what
you eat but how you eat, fostering a deeper
connection with your body and the nourishment
it needs.

Chapter 6
Sustaining Your Ideal Shape

Maintaining your ideal shape is not just about achieving it; it's about sustaining it over time. In this chapter, we'll delve into the strategies and mindset needed to sustain your ideal shape for the long term. We'll cover setting realistic goals, tracking progress effectively, and staying motivated even when faced with challenges.

1. Setting Realistic Goals:

A. Understanding Your Body:
Before setting goals, it's crucial to understand your body's unique needs, limitations, and potential. Consider factors such as your

metabolism, body type, and any medical conditions that may impact your journey.

B. **SMART Goals**:

Set Specific, Measurable, Achievable, Relevant, and Time-bound goals. For example, instead of saying "I want to lose weight," a SMART goal would be "I aim to lose 1-2 pounds per week by following a balanced diet and exercising five days a week for the next three months."

C. **Break It Down**:

Divide your long-term goals into smaller, manageable milestones. This makes your journey less daunting and allows you to celebrate achievements along the way, keeping you motivated.

D. **Be Flexible**:

While it's essential to have goals, it's equally crucial to remain flexible and adjust them as needed. Life can be unpredictable, and your goals may need to adapt accordingly.

2. Tracking Progress

A. Keep a Journal:

Maintain a food and exercise journal to track your daily intake and activities. This helps you identify patterns, triggers, and areas for improvement.

B. Use Technology:

Leverage technology tools like fitness apps, wearable devices, or spreadsheets to track your progress accurately. These tools often provide insights into your calorie intake, macronutrient distribution, and physical activity levels.

C. Measure More Than Weight:

While weight can be a useful indicator, it's not the only measure of progress. Track other metrics like body measurements, body fat percentage, energy levels, and mood to get a comprehensive view of your journey.

D. Regular Assessments:

Schedule regular assessments (weekly or monthly) to evaluate your progress objectively. Reflect on what's working well and what needs adjustment to stay on track.

3. Staying Motivated

A. Find Your Why:

Identify your reasons for wanting to sustain your ideal shape. Whether it's improving health, boosting confidence, or setting a positive example for loved ones, having a strong "why" keeps you motivated during challenging times.

B. Visualize Success:

Create a mental image of yourself achieving your goals. Visualization techniques can reinforce your commitment and drive by making your desired outcome feel more attainable.

C. Celebrate Achievements:

Acknowledge and celebrate every milestone, no matter how small. Whether it's fitting into a smaller size of clothing or completing a challenging workout, each achievement boosts your confidence and motivation.

D. Seek Support:

Surround yourself with a supportive network of friends, family, or online communities who share similar goals. Having a support system can provide encouragement, accountability, and practical advice when facing obstacles.

E. Practice Self-Compassion:

Understand that setbacks are a natural part of the journey. Practice self-compassion and concentrate on your progress rather than perfection rather than being harsh with yourself. Take lessons from failures and turn them into chances to improve.

By setting realistic goals, tracking your progress diligently, and staying motivated through the ups and downs, you can sustain your ideal shape for the long term. Remember that it's not just about reaching your destination but also about enjoying the journey and embracing the positive changes along the way.

Chapter 7
Recipes for Balanced Bites

In this chapter, we'll explore a variety of recipes that are not only delicious but also help you maintain your ideal shape by providing balanced nutrition for breakfast, lunch, dinner, and snacks.

1. Breakfast Ideas

A. Avocado and Egg Breakfast Bowl:

Ingredients:

- 1 ripe avocado
- 2 eggs
- Salt and pepper to taste

- Optional toppings: diced tomatoes, chopped cilantro, salsa

Instructions:

✓ Halve the avocado and scoop out the pit. To make a bigger well, scoop out a little bit more avocado.

✓ Crack an egg into each avocado half.

✓ Season with salt and pepper.

✓ Bake in the oven at 375°F (190°C) for 15-20 minutes or until the eggs are cooked to your desired level of doneness.

✓ Serve hot, topped with diced tomatoes, chopped cilantro, or salsa if desired.

Nutritional Benefits:

✓ Avocados provide healthy fats.

✓ Eggs offer high-quality protein, making this breakfast bowl a satisfying and nutritious option to start your day.

B. Quinoa Breakfast Porridge:

Ingredients:

- 1/2 cup quinoa, rinsed
-One cup of almond milk, or any other type of milk.
- 1 tablespoon honey or maple syrup
- 1/2 teaspoon cinnamon

- Fresh fruit for topping (such as berries, sliced bananas, or diced apples)
- Nuts or seeds for topping (such as chopped almonds or pumpkin seeds)

Instructions:

✓ In a saucepan, combine quinoa, almond milk, honey or maple syrup, and cinnamon.

✓ Bring to a boil, then reduce heat to low and simmer for 15-20 minutes, or until quinoa is cooked and the mixture thickens to a porridge-like consistency, stirring occasionally.

✓ Serve hot, topped with fresh fruit and nuts or seeds.

Nutritional Benefits:

Quinoa is a complete protein, rich in fiber and various vitamins and minerals. Paired with almond milk and fruit, this porridge provides a balanced mix of carbohydrates, protein, and healthy fats.

C. Greek Yogurt Parfait:

Ingredients:

- 1 cup Greek yogurt
- 1/2 cup granola
-Half a cup of mixed berries, including blueberries, raspberries, and strawberries.
- One tablespoon (optional) of maple syrup or honey.

Instructions:

✓ In a serving glass or bowl, layer Greek yogurt, granola, and mixed berries.

✓ Until all of the ingredients are utilized, keep topping.

✓ Drizzle honey or maple syrup on top if desired.

Nutritional Benefits:

✓ Greek yogurt is high in protein and probiotics.

✓ Granola provides fiber and healthy carbohydrates.

✓ Berries are rich in antioxidants, vitamins, and minerals, making this parfait a nutritious and satisfying breakfast option.

D. Spinach and Feta Omelette:

Ingredients:

- 2 eggs
- 1 cup fresh spinach leaves, chopped
- 2 tablespoons crumbled feta cheese
- Salt and pepper to taste
- Cooking spray or olive oil for coating the pan.

Instructions:

✓ Beat the eggs in a bowl until thoroughly combined. Add pepper and salt for seasoning.

✓ Heat a non-stick skillet over medium heat and lightly grease with cooking spray or olive oil.

✓ Pour the beaten eggs into the skillet, tilting the pan to spread them evenly.

✓ Cook for 2-3 minutes, or until the edges start to set.

✓ Evenly top half of the omelet with chopped spinach and crumbled feta cheese.

✓ Fold the other half of the omelet over the filling and cook for another 2-3 minutes, or until the eggs are cooked through.

✓ Transfer the omelet to a platter and enjoy it warm.

Nutritional Benefits:

✓ Spinach is packed with vitamins and minerals.

✓ Eggs provide high-quality protein.

✓ Feta cheese adds a creamy texture and tangy flavor, making this omelet both delicious and nutritious.

E. Whole Wheat Banana Pancakes:

Ingredients:

- 1 ripe banana, mashed

- 1 egg

- 1/2 cup whole wheat flour

- 1/2 cup milk of your choice

- 1 tablespoon honey or maple syrup

- 1/2 teaspoon baking powder

- 1/2 teaspoon vanilla extract

- Pinch of salt

- Coat the pan with butter or cooking spray.

Instructions:

✓ In a bowl, combine mashed banana, egg, whole wheat flour, milk, honey or maple syrup, baking powder, vanilla extract, and salt. Mix until smooth.

✓ Apply a thin layer of frying spray or butter to a nonstick skillet or griddle before heating it to medium heat.

✓ For each pancake, add roughly 1/4 cup of batter to the griddle.

✓ Cook for 2-3 minutes, or until bubbles form on the surface of the pancake.

✓ Flip and cook for another 1-2 minutes, or until golden brown on both sides.

✓ Repeat with the remaining batter.

✓ Serve hot, topped with additional sliced banana, a drizzle of honey or maple syrup, and a sprinkle of cinnamon if desired.

Nutritional Benefits:

✓ These pancakes are made with whole wheat flour, which provides fiber and essential nutrients.

✓ Bananas add natural sweetness and potassium.

✓ Eggs contribute protein, making this breakfast both wholesome and filling.

2. Lunch and Dinner Recipes

In this section, we'll explore satisfying and nutritious recipes for both lunch and dinner that will help you maintain your ideal shape.

A. **Grilled Chicken Salad with Avocado Dressing**:

Ingredients:

- 2 boneless, skinless chicken breasts

- 6 cups mixed salad greens

- 1 cup cherry tomatoes, halved

- 1 cucumber, sliced

- 1/4 red onion, thinly sliced

- 1 avocado, diced

- 2 tablespoons olive oil

- 1 tablespoon lemon juice

- 1 clove garlic, minced

- Salt and pepper to taste

Instructions:

✓ Turn the grill's power to medium-high. Add salt and pepper to chicken breasts for flavor.

✓ Cook the chicken for an overall duration of 6 to 8 minutes on all sides beneath the grill. After five minutes of taking a break, chop.

✓ In a large bowl, combine salad greens, cherry tomatoes, cucumber, red onion, and diced avocado.

✓ In a small bowl, whisk together olive oil, lemon juice, garlic, salt, and pepper to make the dressing.

✓ Drizzle dressing over the salad and toss to coat.

✓ Divide salad among plates and top with sliced grilled chicken.

Nutritional Benefits:

This salad is packed with lean protein from the grilled chicken and healthy fats from the avocado, making it a satisfying and nutritious option for lunch or dinner.

B. **Quinoa Stuffed Bell Peppers:**

Ingredients:

- 4 bell peppers, any color
- One can fifteen ounces of black beans, rinsed and drained.
- One cup of corn kernels, preferably fresh, frozen, or dried.

- 1 cup corn kernels (fresh, frozen, or canned)

- 1 cup diced tomatoes

- 1/2 cup shredded cheddar cheese

- 1 teaspoon chili powder

- 1/2 teaspoon cumin

- Salt and pepper to taste

- Fresh cilantro for garnish (optional)

Instructions:

✓ Raise the oven to 190°C, or 375°F. Chop the tops off of the bell peppers and get rid of the seeds and membranes.

✓ In a large bowl, combine cooked quinoa, black beans, corn, diced tomatoes, shredded cheese, chili powder, cumin, salt, and pepper.

✓ Spoon the quinoa mixture evenly into the bell peppers.

✓ Place the stuffed peppers in a baking dish and cover with foil.

✓ Bake the peppers for 25 to 30 minutes, or until they become tender.

✓ Remove foil and bake for an additional 5 minutes, or until the cheese is melted and bubbly.

✓ Garnish with fresh cilantro if desired before serving.

Nutritional Benefits:

These stuffed bell peppers are packed with protein, fiber, and essential nutrients from quinoa, black beans, and vegetables, making them a healthy and satisfying meal option.

C. **Salmon and Vegetable Stir-Fry**:

Ingredients:

-Two filets of salmon.

– Two tablespoons of soy sauce.

- 1 tablespoon honey

- 1 tablespoon rice vinegar

- 1 teaspoon sesame oil

- 2 cloves garlic, minced

- 1 teaspoon grated ginger

- 2 cups mixed vegetables (such as broccoli, bell peppers, snap peas)

- Cooked brown rice for serving

- Sesame seeds for garnish (optional)

- Sliced green onions for garnish (optional)

Instructions:

✓ In a small bowl, whisk together soy sauce, honey, rice vinegar, sesame oil, minced garlic, and grated ginger to make the sauce. Set aside.

✓ Heat a large skillet or wok over medium-high heat. Add the salmon filets and cook for 3-4 minutes per side, or until cooked through. Remove from the skillet and set aside.

✓ In the same skillet, add mixed vegetables and stir-fry for 4-5 minutes, or until crisp-tender.

✓ Return the cooked salmon to the skillet and pour the sauce over the salmon and vegetables.

Cook for an additional 1-2 minutes, stirring gently to coat everything evenly.

✓ Serve hot cooked brown rice, garnished with sesame seeds and sliced green onions if desired.

Nutritional Benefits:

This stir-fry is rich in omega-3 fatty acids from salmon and packed with vitamins and minerals from mixed vegetables, making it a flavorful and nutritious meal option for lunch or dinner.

D. Lentil and Vegetable Soup

Ingredients:

- One tablespoon of olive oil
- 1 onion, chopped

- 2 carrots, diced

- 2 celery stalks, diced

- 2 cloves garlic, minced

- 1 cup dried green lentils, rinsed

- 4 cups vegetable broth

- 1 can (14 ounces) diced tomatoes

- 1 teaspoon dried thyme

- 1 teaspoon dried oregano

- Salt and pepper to taste

- Fresh parsley for garnish (optional)

Instructions:

✓ In a large pot, heat olive oil over medium heat. Add chopped onion, diced carrots, diced celery, and minced garlic. Cook for 5-6 minutes, or until vegetables are softened.

✓ Add rinsed lentils, vegetable broth, diced tomatoes (with their juices), dried thyme, and dried oregano to the pot. Season with salt and pepper.

✓ Bring the soup to a boil, then reduce heat to low and simmer for 25-30 minutes, or until lentils are tender.

✓ Taste and adjust seasoning if necessary.

✓ Serve hot, garnished with fresh parsley if desired.

Nutritional Benefits:
This hearty lentil and vegetable soup is rich in fiber, protein, and essential nutrients, making it a

satisfying and nourishing option for lunch or dinner.

E. Turkey and Veggie Lettuce Wraps:

Ingredients:

- 1 tablespoon olive oil

- 1 pound ground turkey

- 1 onion, chopped

- 2 cloves garlic, minced

- 1 bell pepper, diced

- 1 zucchini, diced

- 1 carrot, grated

- 1/4 cup hoisin sauce

- 2 tablespoons soy sauce

- 1 teaspoon sesame oil

- Butter lettuce leaves, for serving

- Sliced green onions for garnish (optional)

- Sesame seeds for garnish (optional)

Instructions:

✓ In a sizable skillet over medium heat, warm up the olive oil. Break up the ground turkey with a spoon while it cooks until it appears brown.

✓ Add chopped onion and minced garlic to the skillet and cook for 2-3 minutes, or until softened.

✓ Stir in diced bell pepper, diced zucchini, and grated carrot. Cook for 5-6 minutes, or until vegetables are tender.

✓ Mix the soy sauce, sesame oil, and hoisin sauce in a small bowl. Over the turkey and vegetable combination in the skillet, pour the sauce. After combining, heat for a further two to three minutes.

✓ Spoon turkey and veggie mixture into butter lettuce leaves to serve. If preferred, garnish with sesame seeds and sliced green onions.

Nutritional Benefits:
These lettuce wraps are low in carbs and packed with lean protein from ground turkey and a variety of vegetables, making them a light yet satisfying option for lunch or dinner.

3. Snack Options

For those mid-day cravings or a quick energy boost

A. Greek Yogurt with Berries and Almonds:

Ingredients:

- 1/2 cup Greek yogurt

- 1/4 cup mixed berries (such as strawberries, blueberries, and raspberries)

- 1 tablespoon sliced almonds

Instructions:

✓ In a small bowl, scoop Greek yogurt.

✓ Top with mixed berries and sliced almonds.

✓ Enjoy this protein-packed snack that provides a balance of carbohydrates, protein, and healthy fats.

Nutritional Benefits:

Greek yogurt offers protein and probiotics, while berries provide fiber and antioxidants. Almonds add crunch and healthy fats, making this snack both delicious and nutritious.

B. Apple Slices with Peanut Butter

Ingredients:

- 1 apple, sliced
- Two tablespoons of peanut butter (or a different type of nut or seed butter)

Instructions:

✓ Slice the apple into thin wedges.

✓ On each apple slice, spread a little peanut butter.

✓ Enjoy this simple yet satisfying snack that combines sweet and savory flavors.

Nutritional Benefits:

Apples are rich in fiber and vitamins, while peanut butter provides protein and healthy fats, making this snack a perfect combination of crunch and creaminess.

C. Hummus and Veggie Sticks:

Ingredients:

- 1/4 cup hummus

- Assorted vegetable sticks (such as carrot, cucumber, bell pepper, and celery)

Instructions:

✓ Place hummus in a small bowl.

✓ Cut assorted vegetables into sticks or slices.

✓ Dip vegetable sticks into hummus and enjoy this crunchy and satisfying snack.

Nutritional Benefits:

Hummus is a good source of plant-based protein and fiber, while vegetables offer vitamins, minerals, and additional fiber, making this snack both nutritious and filling.

D. Trail Mix:

Ingredients:

- 1/4 cup nuts (such as almonds, cashews, or walnuts)
- 1/4 cup dried fruit (such as raisins, cranberries, or apricots)
- Two teaspoons of solid or chipped dark chocolate
- 2 tablespoons pumpkin seeds or sunflower seeds

Instructions:

✓ In a small bowl, combine nuts, dried fruit, dark chocolate chips, and seeds.

✓ Mix well and portion into individual servings for a convenient grab-and-go snack option.

Nutritional Benefits:
This trail mix provides a mix of protein, healthy fats, and carbohydrates, along with vitamins, minerals, and antioxidants from nuts, dried fruit, seeds, and dark chocolate, making it a satisfying and nutritious snack.

E. **Rice Cake with Avocado and Tomato**:

Ingredients:

- 1 rice cake
- 1/4 ripe avocado, mashed
- 1 small tomato, sliced

- Pinch of salt and pepper (optional)

Instructions:

✓ Spread mashed avocado evenly on top of the rice cake.

✓ Arrange tomato slices on top of the avocado.

✓ Sprinkle with a pinch of salt and pepper if desired.

✓ Enjoy this crunchy and creamy snack that's packed with flavor and nutrients.

Nutritional Benefits:
Rice cakes provide a crunchy base, while avocado offers healthy fats and tomatoes add

freshness and vitamins, making this snack both light and satisfying.

Experiment with different combinations and flavors to find your favorites. Enjoy!

Conclusion

In the journey towards achieving and sustaining your ideal shape, "Balanced Bites: A Guide to Sustaining Your Ideal Shape" has provided a comprehensive roadmap, emphasizing the significance of balance, moderation, and mindful eating. By understanding the principles of nutrition, portion control, and the importance of physical activity, readers have been equipped with the tools necessary to make informed decisions about their health and wellness.Throughout this guide, we've explored the concept of balance not only in terms of food choices but also in how we approach our lifestyle. By emphasizing the importance of incorporating a variety of nutrient-dense foods, enjoying treats in moderation, and cultivating a positive relationship with food, readers have been encouraged to adopt sustainable habits that support long-term health and well-being.

Moreover, "Balanced Bites" has highlighted the significance of listening to our bodies and honoring their signals. By practicing mindful eating techniques such as paying attention to hunger and fullness cues, savoring each bite, and eating with intention, readers have learned to foster a deeper connection with the food they consume and the impact it has on their overall health.As we conclude this journey, it's essential to recognize that achieving and maintaining our ideal shape is not solely about the number on the scale or fitting into a certain clothing size. True wellness encompasses physical, mental, and emotional well-being, and it's a journey that requires patience, self-compassion, and a willingness to embrace imperfection.

In closing, "Balanced Bites: A Guide to Sustaining Your Ideal Shape" serves as a valuable resource for anyone seeking to cultivate a healthier relationship with food, achieve their ideal shape, and sustain it for the long term. By implementing the principles outlined in this guide, readers have the power to transform their lives and embrace a lifestyle of balance, vitality, and self-care. Remember, it's not about perfection, but rather progress, and every step towards a healthier you is worth celebrating. Here's to your journey towards balanced living and a happier, healthier you.